HIS &

HERS

THE LITTLE BOOK OF
INTIMACY

SHARON PLATT-MCDONALD
MSC, RHV, RM, RGN

Copyright © 2011

First Published 2011

ISBN number: 978-1-907244-12-4

British Library Cataloguing in Publication Data.
A catalogue record for this book is available
from the British Library.

All Bible quotations not attributed to the New
King James Version or the New International
Version come from the King James Version, with
a single exception from the Clear Word Bible.

Published by
Autumn House Publishing (Europe) Ltd,

Alma Park, Grantham, Lincolnshire, England.

Design: Abigail Murphy

Printed in Thailand

INTRODUCTION

While completing an MSc in Health Sciences at St George's Medical School, London, I opted for a module on behavioural science. Most of my fellow students already had an idea of what constitutes 'normal' or 'abnormal' eating and sleeping patterns, but there was controversy over what constituted 'normality' in terms of sexuality.

Realising that variations in religious observance, culture, age and gender all affect our perception and practice of sexual norms, the class concluded that the phrase 'normal' straddles a wide range on the spectrum of human behaviour.

I got married two weeks after I graduated from this course, which gave me a lot of food for thought!

In this little book of intimacy we look at gender-specific behaviours, communication styles and information processing, as well as male and female expressions of love, and the health implications of sexual intimacy.

GENDER DIFFERENCES

'And he answered and said unto them,
Have ye not read, that he which made
them at the beginning made them male
and female . . . ?' *(Matthew 19:4)*

You may have read the book, *Men are from Mars, Women are from Venus*. If so, you would have concluded that gender differences are quite significant. A large body of scientific evidence exists that highlights the psychological, physiological and sexual differences between men and women. In this section, we compare and contrast some of these differences in the areas of communication, emotional response, and romantic and sexual expression.

COMMUNICATION DIFFERENCES

⊙ Men tend to talk less than women, using approximately 7,000 words a day on average, as opposed to women's 20,000 words.

⊙ Key conversation topics for men include the latest technology, sports, news, politics, music and women – typical topics for women include relationships, plans, health, food, clothes and family matters.

⊙ Men tend to be more factual, whereas women express their feelings.

⊙ Men tend to solve problems independently, engaging in solo activities to process information. Women, on the other hand, need to talk through their problems and seek connections with others.

⊙ Men are solution-orientated, whereas women discuss issues in order to be heard.

⊙ Men have a dominant hemisphere which they use for language, usually the left side of the brain. By contrast, women do not favour one hemisphere over another.

⊙ Generally, boys develop conversational skills after girls do. MRI scans reveal that the *corpus callosum*, which regulates communication between the brain's two hemispheres, is larger in females.

EMOTIONAL RESPONSE

The differences between the ways in which
men and women express their thoughts,
feelings and emotions can influence their
emotional well-being
and relationships. The Mind Survey
found the following variations between
the genders in their communication
of feelings and emotions:

⊙ Men were half as likely as women to talk about their problems with their friends.

⊙ Men were less likely to express emotion: women were five times more likely to feel tearful.

⊙ 45% of men reported believing that they could fight their emotions, compared with only 36% of women.

⊙ 4% of men aged 18-24 would see a counsellor if they felt depressed, compared with 13% of women of the same age.

⊙ If they felt depressed for longer than two weeks, 23% of men would see their GP, but women reported that they were more likely to seek medical advice.

⊙ The brain's limbic system, responsible for emotions and bonding, is larger in females. Consequently, women create bonds more easily, are more expressive, and are more in touch with their feelings; on the other hand, men are less at risk of depression, particularly during periods of significant hormonal change, than women are.

SEXUAL RESPONSE AND EXPRESSION

⊙ Men are more sexually motivated than women from the onset of puberty; however, women become more sexually motivated as they develop confidence in their sexuality.

⊙ Men are usually visually stimulated; some women are visually stimulated too, but emotional, romantic and relational issues are equally as important.

⊙ Men usually deepen their emotional connection through sexual intimacy; whereas women usually seek emotional connection as a precursor to sexual intimacy.

⊙ Men tend to view sexual intimacy as an expression of love, whereas women generally want to experience love before expressing sexual intimacy.

- Often, following an argument, men want to make love in order to make up, whereas women need to make up before making love.

- Anger does not necessarily impair sexual desire in men, but it usually does in women.

⊙ In men, sexual withdrawal has been linked with damaging developmental experiences. In women, it has commonly been related to negative emotions.

⊙ Men sometimes watch a film or some sport after lovemaking, or fall asleep, but women often want 'pillow talk' and cuddles.

⊙ Young men long for sexual fulfilment, whereas young women commonly place love and romance before sexual fulfilment.

⊙ Research on the religious beliefs and sexuality of men found that there was no correlation between church attendance and sexual desire. Women who attend church are less likely to have permissive attitudes about sex.

MALE TALK
— WHAT MEN WANT

Much research and analysis has been
undertaken to determine what men want.
Here is a list of some of the most
commonly-expressed traits which
men expect in a woman:

◉ Fun and excitement, good looks, and
great sex (frequent, consistent
and passionate).

⊙ The ability to look after herself, and
femininity, combined with a lack of
aggression or loudness.

⊙ Respect, and the ability to listen,
provide support, and show an interest.

⊙ Confidence, trustworthiness
and a sense of humour.

💟 A Spirit-filled character
(if the man is a Christian).

💟 Similar interests, and an acceptance
of the need to spend some time
alone and with male friends.

⊙ Gentleness and kindness.

⊙ Commitment, domestic skills, and the willingness to be there for a man at the end of the day and share a meal with him.

FEMALE TALK
– WHAT WOMEN WANT

One survey, entitled 'What Women Want',
posed three questions: 1) Do women have
insatiable appetites? 2) Have women's
needs changed? 3) Are women losing their
femininity? In the ensuing debate, men
were left with the feeling that women did
not know what they wanted
and were hard to please.

No agreement was reached as to whether or not women's needs had changed, but both men and women agreed that some women were losing their femininity and becoming more like men. Some women felt that this was because men were losing their masculinity, causing women to become more self-reliant.

The women were asked to identify those
characteristics which they most desired in
a man. They gave these responses:

⦿ Love, romance, attention,
security and commitment.

⦿ A relationship with God
(if the woman is a Christian).

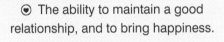

⊙ The ability to maintain a good relationship, and to bring happiness.

⊙ Money, honesty, and respect.

MEETING NEEDS

'He who is unmarried cares for the things
of the Lord – how he may please the Lord.
But he who is married cares about the
things of the world – how he may please
his wife. There is [also] a difference
between a wife and a virgin. The unmarried
woman cares about the things of the Lord,
that she may be holy both in body and in
spirit. But she who is married cares about
the things of the world – how she may
please her husband.'

1 Corinthians 7:32-34, NKJV

Before I got married, if you
had asked me how a
husband's needs could be met,
I might have said: 'When he comes
home, his slippers should be by the
door, the table should be laid and the
dinner ready to serve. He'll want to eat a
tasty meal with you while you listen
attentively to him as he talks about his day,
after which you can share a shortened
version of your own day,
being light-hearted so that there will
be no opportunity for headaches
when he says "let's go upstairs" '.

However, with the blurring of gender roles in the West over recent years, and with the competing agendas which some have in relationships, there are still divergent views on the struggle to understand the opposite sex.

HIS NEEDS, HER NEEDS

I was once asked to preside at the wedding reception of a friend. In preparation for the role, I did some research on men and women's expectations of marriage. I came across an interesting quotation: 'The man decides on the landscape; the woman sets the climate.'

It was interesting to examine a potential marriage landscape: the environment in which love is nurtured or neglected, in which needs are met or left unmet. What would be the impact on the landscape if the climate were not favourable, or vice versa?

To some extent, marriages which experience 'extreme climates', or 'harsh environments', usually contain selfishness, unmet needs and misunderstanding. In *His Needs, Her Needs*, Dr Willard Harley presents the ways in which gender needs are expressed; as well as the need for both husbands and wives to understand each other's needs, to feel comfortable expressing their own needs, and to feel that their needs are being met.

Dr Harley identified five of the most
basic needs, for both husbands
and wives, in any marriage:

MALE NEEDS: Sexual fulfilment;
Recreational companionship;
An attractive spouse;
Domestic support; and Admiration.

FEMALE NEEDS: Affection; Conversation;
Honesty and openness; Financial support;
and Family commitment.

RELATIONSHIPS AND INTIMACY

'The LORD God said, "It is not good for the man to be alone. I will make a helper suitable for him." ' *(Genesis 2:18, NIV)*

God knew of our need to form relationships with like-minded people. Although in its original context the passage of Scripture on the preceding page referred specifically to Adam, it can apply equally well to both genders – both men and women can be blessed by relationships.

Spiritual, emotional, physical and sexual intimacy is key to a successful relationship.

You may have heard one definition of the word 'intimacy' as 'into-me-see'. Individuals who become intimate with each other become vulnerable. We expose our emotions, our inner selves, to each other, connecting with each other and meeting each other's needs.

SPIRITUAL CONNECTION

A spiritual connection encompasses the beliefs, moral values, and behaviours in a relationship. A spiritually compatible relationship has God at its centre, and promotes a union which builds each person's connection with God. Shared core beliefs, expressed in a nurturing environment, are essential to the long-term survival of a couple's relationship.

Sometimes we face challenges to all that we believe and hold dear. In these times, a shared belief in God will smooth the way and help to solidify your relationship. What level of spiritual support do you give to each other? How would you like your spouse to help you further? How can you offer better support to your spouse?

After a hard day at work, my husband would come home and share the events of the day with me. Interestingly enough, these would be the very days upon which I felt particularly impressed to pray for him. Whenever I tell him that I have been praying for him during the day, he says, 'I know. I felt your prayers'.

On the facing page are some measures that my husband and I found beneficial:

SPECIAL DAYS OF
FASTING AND PRAYER.
We usually fast for half a day on
a weekly basis. Sometimes it is for
something specific; other times we
just use that time to thank God.

TEXT MESSAGES, with promise Scriptures or
inspirational quotations, that we send to
each other to bless each other.

AUDIBLE AFFIRMATIONS AND BLESSINGS.
My husband often places his hands on my
head and offers a spontaneous prayer or
blessing over me. Sometimes he just
speaks into my life words of encouragement
or passages of Scripture relating to God's
promises. I do the same for him.

EMOTIONAL INTIMACY

'Come now, and let us reason together,
saith the LORD . . .' *(Isaiah 1:18)*

Behavioural scientists agree that
within the communication process . . .

. . . these are generally four key elements:

- ⦿ What we say.

- ⦿ What we mean.

- ⦿ What we hear.

- ⦿ What we understand.

All of these elements are necessary in the marital relationship. When we are unsure of what is being said, it is helpful to seek clarity before drawing conclusions. Your marriage partner will feel appreciated and understood. This will strengthen your marriage.

EMOTIONAL BONDING
AND THE EXPRESSION OF LOVE

'Her husband has full confidence in her
and lacks nothing of value.'
(Proverbs 31:11, NIV)

The Bible emphasises the connection and
the trust which exist between husband and
wife in an ideal marital relationship. Men
need to have confidence
in their wives.

'Scarcely had I passed them when I found
the one my heart loves. I held him
and would not let him go. . .'
(Song of Solomon 3:4, NIV)

It is important for both marriage partners to
feel emotionally connected. Women in
particular seek emotional bonding
and closeness.

LOVE LANGUAGE

Dr Gary Chapman, author of *The Five Love Languages*, writes about the importance of being able to express your love in a way your spouse can understand. This, he feels, is possible using types of communication which he calls 'love languages', identifying them as:

⊙ WORDS OF AFFIRMATION (which boost your spouse's confidence)

⊙ QUALITY TIME (giving undivided attention to your spouse, having fun together)

⦿ GIFTS (the giving of which symbolises
your fondness for each other)

⦿ ACTS OF SERVICE (practical ways in
which you may help each other)

⦿ PHYSICAL TOUCH (holding hands,
hugging, kissing, stroking
each other's back)

Which love language do you speak? Which
love language does your partner
understand? Do you appreciate your
partner's love language?

PHYSICAL INTIMACY:
THE POWER OF TOUCH

Hugging is generally used to express affection, appreciation, happiness or non-sexual love. Women in particular value non-sexual touching. It helps them feel connected and valued, and provides reassurance. For some it is both soothing and affirming, giving them a feeling of warmth and security. Some women appreciate hugs more than others.

Men, however, often touch in a different way. Observe men in a group setting, and you will notice that their touches are more solid and heavy: back slaps, punches and firm handshakes are their primary mode of communication. Generally speaking, men understand soft, gentle touches to have sexual overtones. Touching in a gentle manner can, in some contexts, cause men to feel vulnerable, dependent or even threatened.

SEXUAL INTIMACY

The biblical account of sexual expression found in the Song of Solomon is not something often discussed in a Sabbath sermon. However, it is enlightening, and couples can read it together to enhance their verbal expression of love.

While the King James
Version flows with poetic expression,
modern translations bring a
more direct message:

'How beautiful and pleasing you are! How
pure are the delights of your love! You are
as graceful and tall as a palm tree. Your
breasts are like clusters of dates. I will
climb the palm tree and take hold of its
fruit. Your breasts are like clusters of
ripened grapes. Your breath is like the
fragrance of ripened apples and the taste
of your lips like freshly squeezed juice.'
(Song of Solomon 7:6-8,
The Clear Word Bible)

SEXUAL DESIRE

Sexual desire or drive is
referred to by the term 'libido'.
Libido varies from person to person.
Hormonal influences are at the heart of
sexual desire. Oestrogen and testosterone
are the hormones which account for
most of the differences between
men and women.

During lovemaking, the hormone called
'oxytocin' is released, at the point of
orgasm, by both the man and the woman –
this heightens sexual pleasure.

Another hormone, vasopressin, is secreted
as the man becomes aroused.
It is linked to the male drive for
sexual expression.

Sexual motivation is influenced to some degree in both men and women by thoughts and feelings. However, men's sexual arousal and desire tend to be more spontaneous than the arousal of women, whose sexual 'triggers' are often more to do with how the man and woman relate to each other. Women value emotional connection as the key to sexual desire. They are influenced by social and cultural factors as well.

Generally speaking, a man's sex drive peaks in his early 20s, and a woman's in her late 30s – sometimes even in her 40s.

Dr Edward Laumann,
professor of sociology at
the University of Chicago, says:
'Sexual desire in women is extremely
sensitive to environment and context.'
It seems that candles and scents (and a
willingness by her husband to help out with
the housework) can make the
night more enjoyable!

Esther Perel writes: 'For women, there is a
need for a plot – hence the romantic novel.
It is more about the anticipation, how you
get there; it is the longing
that is the fuel for desire.'

By contrast, however, men appear not to
need as much imagination.

LOW LIBIDO

For some spouses, the words 'not tonight, darling' become a frequent response to the prospect of sexual intimacy. There are many reasons for a reduced libido:

- ⊙ Alcohol, medication or low testosterone levels

- ⊙ Depression, sleep deprivation or stress

- ⊙ Erectile dysfunction, obesity, or a lack of confidence in one's own body

- ⊙ Lack of emotional intimacy, the onset of menopause, or family commitments.

FREQUENCY

'Unlike vitamins, there are no daily requirements [for the frequency of sex]', said Weiner Davis in *The Sex-Starved Marriage*. 'If both spouses are satisfied with having a sex-lite marriage, that's great. However, it's much more often the case that couples are polarised, that one person is unhappy with the quality and quantity of their sex life and the other is saying, "What's the big deal? Get a life." '

Only 40% of married couples admitted being very satisfied with their sex lives when Weiner Davis interviewed them. Medical problems and medications (such as antidepressants and contraceptives) can sometimes cause a decrease in sexual desire.

WHAT DOES
THE RESEARCH SHOW?

⊙ One in five married couples has
intercourse fewer than ten times a year.

⊙ One in three married couples struggles
with the problem of mismatched sexual
desire. This is the main reason that
couples seek counselling.

⦿ Working long hours or desperately searching for jobs can cause fatigue and stress, making matters worse.

⦿ The average married couple has sex once or twice a week.

HEALTH BENEFITS
OF SEXUAL INTERCOURSE

It's official – good sex can
enhance your overall health!

Scientists have identified ten key health
benefits of regular sexual intercourse:

⦿ Sex is a calorie-burner. Thirty minutes of
sex burns 85 calories or more. That might
not sound like a lot, but it all adds up. Sex
is a great form of exercise.

⊙ Sex enhances
cardiovascular health.
Contrary to popular opinion,
the energy expended in lovemaking
is not harmful to those with advanced age
or heart conditions. Scientists in the UK
studied 914 men over a twenty-year period.
Their findings, published in the Journal of
Epidemiology and Community Health,
revealed that the frequency of sex was not
associated with their risk of suffering a
stroke. The researchers also found that
those who have sex twice or more each
week are half as likely to suffer a fatal
heart attack as those who have sex
less often than once a month.

⊙ Sex boosts your immunity.
Engaging in intercourse once or
twice each week has been linked with
higher levels of an antibody called
immunoglobulin A (or IgA), which protects
against colds and other infections.
Those who have sex once or twice a
week have the highest levels of IgA.

⊙ Sex improves intimacy and bonding.
An orgasm increases your levels of the
hormone oxytocin, also known as
'the love hormone'. This enhances
bonding and builds trust. Oxytocin
helps us to nurture and to bond.

⊙ Sex improves pain relief.
As oxytocin levels rise, endorphins (the feel-good hormones) also increase. This causes our perception of pain to decline.

⊙ Sex reduces the risk of prostate cancer.
A study, published in the *British Journal of Urology International*, was carried out on the sexual activity of men with and without cancer. The study concluded that frequent ejaculations, especially in men between the ages of 20 and 30, may have reduced their risk of developing prostate cancer later on in life.

⦿ Sex strengthens the pelvic floor muscles. When women undertake pelvic exercises, there are many health benefits. Such exercises strengthen the muscles in that area, preventing urine incontinence later on in life. They also improve sexual pleasure, for the wife as well as for the husband, and can enhance sexual performance. To perform a pelvic exercise, tighten the muscles around the vagina and back passage, lifting them upwards as if trying to stop the passing of water or wind, and keep the muscles taut for between one and five seconds for each contraction. (Men, you can do these exercises in a similar way.)

⊙ Sex boosts self-esteem. One of the 237 reasons people have given for having sex is the boosting of self-esteem. Dr Gina Ogden, a sex therapist and marriage and family therapist, states that, generally, even those who already have high self-esteem sometimes have sex to make themselves feel better.

⊙ Sex helps you sleep better. During an orgasm, the hormone oxytocin is released, which promotes sleep. If you have been wondering why men find it so easy to fall asleep after making love, this is the reason! Sound sleep helps you to maintain a healthy weight and level of blood pressure.

THE FOOD FACTOR

As people enter the middle of their lives,
their sex drive generally decreases in
strength. Several foods are reported to
boost libido, but some foods seem to
reduce it, including saturated fats
(found in fast foods), sugar, and alcohol.
Cutting down on these may
improve your sex drive.

The testosterone levels of both
men and women control their libido.
Zinc and vitamin B are required for
testosterone production, and these are
both found in the foods we eat regularly.
Nutritional deficiency increases with age,
but increasing your intake of foods which
contain both zinc and vitamin B will give
your libido a boost, and provide
other health benefits.

Zinc is lost during an orgasm, but eating zinc-rich foods will help to replenish you. The following foods, when accompanied by a regular exercise programme, can enhance your libido:

⊙ Asparagus is rich in vitamin E, which enables the production of testosterone

⊙ Almonds are rich in essential fatty acids, which enable the production of male hormones

⊙ Avocados are rich in folic acid, which helps your body to metabolise proteins

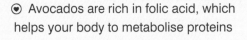 Bananas are rich in potassium, and are a great energy source

- Brown rice is a good source of the zinc needed for testosterone production

- Blueberries are rich in soluble fibre, which moves cholesterol through the digestive system and prevents it from clogging up your arteries. Blueberries also contain compounds that improve circulation, which can result in a natural Viagra-like effect

⊙ Basil is reported to stimulate the sex
drive and boost fertility in women

⊙ Celery is rich in androsterone, a
hormone and pheromone

⊙ Eggs are sources of vitamins B5 and
B6, which help you fight stress and
balance your hormone levels – both of
these effects are crucial for a healthy libido

⦿ Figs are rich in some amino acids which may increase libido; figs are also reported to increase sexual stamina

⦿ Garlic, when it is cut, produces allicin, a chemical that may increase blood-flow to the sexual organs. However, not everyone likes the taste of garlic, so ask your spouse before eating it!

⦿ Ginger rapidly increases the circulation of blood, which benefits your libido

⦿ Honey is rich in vitamin B-complex, which supports both the function of neurotransmitters responsible for sexual arousal and the production of testosterone; honey is also rich in boron, which facilitates the body's use of oestrogen: a hormone that assists blood-flow and arousal.

- Pomegranate juice, when taken over a long period, fights erectile dysfunction

- Oats release testosterone into the blood supply, increasing the strength of both libido and orgasm

- Pine nuts are rich in zinc, which is used in the production of testosterone

⊙ Pumpkin seeds are rich in zinc, which not only aids the production of testosterone but also prevents prostate enlargement and other male sexual health problems

⊙ Spinach is rich in magnesium, which dilates blood vessels – this has a salutary effect on erections.

THE AGE FACTOR

Nancy Better defines a mid-life crisis as 'a time of profound psychological turbulence that usually occurs between the ages of 38 and 55, and often results in dramatic life changes. It can last from 2 to 12 years; the defining symptom is a sense that the values that have guided you for many years no longer hold meaning.'

Hormonal changes such as lowered testosterone levels can cause physical, emotional and sexual changes in men. Going through a mid-life crisis can have an impact upon your marriage.

RECOGNISING A MID-LIFE CRISIS

Frequently reported problems include:

⊙ Sudden changes to sexual behaviour
(either the loss or increase
of sexual appetite)

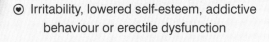 Irritability, lowered self-esteem, addictive
behaviour or erectile dysfunction

⊙ Sudden changes of image,
particularly to look 'youthful'

⊙ Behavioural changes (including secrecy and isolation) or an extra-marital affair

⊙ Depression, lethargy or fatigue (all often otherwise inexplicable)

⊙ Loss of interest in work, family or friends; or the replacement of old friends.

GENDER DIFFERENCES

Nancy Better's research 'shows that women's midlife crises are likely to stem from introspection, a family event, or a problem such as divorce, death or disappointment in their children. Men's midlife crises are more likely to be driven by work or career issues. Even though more women these days are working, I find that these differences haven't entirely disappeared.'

MEDICAL INTERVENTION

It may be necessary to seek medical help if there are significant health or physiological changes. Additionally, if you are emotionally fragile, an assessment may also be useful. There may be underlying physical illnesses linked to the symptoms of a mid-life crisis. For example, erectile dysfunction may be linked to depression, diabetes or heart disease.

THE MENOPAUSE

The menopause is defined as the point at which a woman naturally stops ovulating and ceases menstruation. Menopause occurs when a woman comes to the end of the time when she can reproduce, and her levels of oestrogen and progesterone drop.

'Going through the change' is a common description of what happens to a woman in the middle of her life. Some women go through the menopause without much discomfort and with few obvious changes. However, many women encounter the challenges of annoying symptoms that affect their physical, emotional, sexual and social well-being.

PHYSICAL SYMPTOMS
OF THE MENOPAUSE

- ⊙ Hot flushes, night sweats
  or heart palpitations

- ⊙ Headaches, sleeplessness or fatigue

⊙ Bloating, weight gain or
tenderness of the breasts

⊙ Irregular periods,
vaginal dryness or loss of libido

⊙ Muscle tension, sore joints, urinary
tract infections or frequent urination.

EMOTIONAL OR MENTAL SYMPTOMS OF THE MENOPAUSE

- ⊙ Mood swings, irritability, aggressiveness, sadness, anxiety or depression

- ⊙ Difficulty concentrating or lack of motivation

⦿ Tension

 Lapses or loss of memory.

The menopause is a natural process
that all women experience.

NATURAL INTERVENTIONS IN THE MENOPAUSE

⊙ Maintain a balanced diet. Whole grains, cold pressed oils, leafy vegetables and nuts can help to keep the body healthy and potentially relieve hot flushes. Soy may also ease mild hot flushes. It is best to use a small amount of simply-processed soy products: the natural preparations of tofu, miso and tempeh are healthier than the more popular, processed soy products.

⊙ Consume Omega-3 and Omega-6. These essential fatty acids can help to regulate hormones and combat mood swings. Flax seeds, pumpkin seeds and safflowers are good sources of Omega-3 and Omega-6.

⊙ Ingest vitamin D. This helps to prevent the onset of osteoporosis, a weakening of the bones brought on by the menopause.

⊙ Get lots of calcium. You need this daily to help keep your bones strong.

⊙ Take vitamin B-complex. This vitamin helps you to maintain a healthy nervous system. B-vitamin levels are often depleted by the emotional stress resulting from the menopause. Vitamin B helps your body to perform its proper metabolic functions, and decreases irritability and fatigue.

⊙ Avoid stimulants and toxins. Caffeine, alcohol and cigarettes all magnify the negative effects of the menopause.

⊙ Avoid junk food. Too much salt
and sugar can also magnify the
effects of the menopause.

⊙ Choose foods that are low in
saturated fat and cholesterol.

⊙ Keep active. Exercise releases
endorphins (also known as the
'happy hormones', because they
help to make you feel good).

SUPPORT

Menopausematters.co.uk is an independent, clinician-led website. It provides accessible, up-to-date, accurate information about the menopause, menopausal symptoms, and treatment options, including hormone replacement therapy (HRT) and alternative therapies, so that women and health professionals can make informed choices about how to manage the menopause.

THE A-Z OF INTIMACY

A is for AFFIRMATION. You should always give words of affirmation throughout your marriage to make your partner feel encouraged.

A is also ANGER AVOIDANCE. Deal with anger promptly; avoid bickering, especially at bedtime.

' " In your anger do not sin": Do not let the sun go down while you are still angry'
(Ephesians 4:26, NIV)

B is for BLESSINGS. Blessing your spouse has both spiritual and emotional benefits. When this is done audibly, it also helps to affirm your spouse as well, creating an atmosphere in which the Presence of God is felt.

'I will bless her and will surely give you a son by her. I will bless her so that she will be the mother of nations; kings of peoples will come from her.' *(Genesis 17:16, NIV)*

B

C is for COMMUNICATION. Good communication starts with good conversation; you should listen carefully to make sure you understand and know how to respond to one another.

'Come now, and let us reason together, saith the LORD' *(Isaiah 1:18)*

'A soft answer turns away wrath,
But a harsh word stirs up anger.'
(Proverbs 15:1, NKJV)

C is also for CONFLICT RESOLUTION.
It is crucial for married couples to find
amicable, friendly ways in which to resolve
their conflicts. You should try to avoid
heated arguments and ongoing
misunderstandings, if you want to nurture
your relationship. Forgive each other, trust
each other, and handle your emotions
appropriately, in order to handle conflict
effectively when it comes.

'. . . seek peace and pursue it.'
(1 Peter 3:11, NKJV)

C

C is also for COMMITMENT.
How beautiful it is to see
couples still together, at a ripe old age,
celebrating fifty years and more of
marriage! Commitment includes staying
true to your marital vows, and resolving to
make them work even when things are
difficult. Seek ways in which you can build
your relationship, overcome barriers and
grow your love for one another.

'. . . Have ye not read, that he which made
them at the beginning made them male
and female, and said, For this cause shall a
man leave father and mother, and shall
cleave to his wife: and they twain shall be
one flesh?' *(Matthew 19:4, 5)*

C

D is for DESIRE.
So many things can spark
your desire for your spouse:

⊙ Your spouse's words

⊙ Your spouse's hairstyle,
clothing or eye contact

⊙ The scent of your spouse, or of
perfume, cologne or scented candles

⊙ Intimate thoughts or touches,
and an appropriate ambience

'Turn your eyes from me; they overwhelm
me. Your hair is like a flock of goats
descending from Gilead'!
(Song of Solomon 6:5, NIV)

D

D is also for DATES:
You can keep your relationship sparkling by going out on a date together – or even by staying in together! The key is to take work off the schedule and give your undivided attention to each other, whether it be on a date night or a family weekend. This specially protected time gives you something to look forward to and value as the relationship bond is strengthened.

'Come with me from Lebanon, my bride, come with me from Lebanon. Descend from the crest of Armana, from the top of Senir, the summit of Hermon . . .'
(Song of Solomon 4:8, NIV)

E is for EFFORT. In a discussion on marriage some time ago, a senior church member advised: 'Marriage is like a job that you work at every day; you have to put the effort in'.

How much effort do you put into making your marriage a success? Marriage retreats, courses, relationship books and so on are all resources to be made use of on your journey together.

'Dear children, let us not love with words or tongue but with actions and in truth.'
(1 John 3:18, NIV)

E is also for EMOTIONS.
In a marital relationship,
spouses feel responsible for each
other's happiness, as they now have
their spouse's emotions as well
as their own to consider.

Developing a positive outlook can build
emotional resilience. Identifying the
emotional triggers that affect your
relationship, both positively and negatively,
will enable you and your spouse to work
through them as you understand and
support each other.

'When my heart was grieved and my spirit
embittered, I was senseless and ignorant; I
was a beast before you.'
(Psalm 73:21, 22, NIV)

F is for FAITHFULNESS.
Any sexual intimacy which
occurs outside the marriage
relationship breaks the marital
covenant and has dire consequences.

One repercussion is the damaging of
self-esteem, particularly in the offended
spouse; it makes him or her feel
replaceable, sexually inadequate
and not special.

'Let your fountain be blessed,
And rejoice with the wife of your youth. . . .
For why should you, my son, be
enraptured by an immoral woman,
And be embraced in the arms of a
seductress?'
(Proverbs 5:18, 20, NKJV)

F

F is also for FORGIVENESS.
To forgive someone is to let
go of resentment and to untie yourself from
thoughts and feelings about the offence.

Those closest to us are the ones we have
to forgive most often. Forgiveness is a
natural consequence of love. When we
forgive an individual, we are extending love
to that person, just as Christ extends his
love to us in his forgiveness of our sins.
Forgiveness promotes inner peace,
deepens our spiritual experience and
makes us more Christlike.

'For if you forgive men their trespasses,
your heavenly Father will also forgive you.'
(Matthew 6:14, NKJV)

G is for GIFTS. Gifts do not
have to be expensive; the act of
giving a gift sends a powerful message
of love to your spouse. When birthdays
and anniversaries are remembered through
the giving of gifts, your spouse will feel
loved and not neglected.

'But thou shalt go unto my country, and to
my kindred, and take a wife unto my son
Isaac. . . . And the servant brought forth
jewels of silver, and jewels of gold, and
raiment, and gave them to Rebekah: he
gave also to her brother and to her mother
precious things.' *(Genesis 24:4, 53)*

G

H is for HUGS. There is a correlation between the amount of hugs a woman receives and the lowness of her blood pressure. Hugs increase levels of oxytocin, a hormone associated with bonding and building trust. Hug every day to boost both your love relationship and your health.

'His left hand is under my head, and his right hand doth embrace me.'
(Song of Solomon 2:6)

H is also for HUMOUR. Laughter aids in the release of endorphins ('happy hormones'). Don't take life too seriously! Learn to appreciate the lighter side of life; enjoy fun activities together which make you both laugh, as this will nurture your relationship, keeping it fresh and vibrant.

'A merry heart makes a cheerful countenance,
But by sorrow of the heart the spirit is broken.' *(Proverbs 15:13, NKJV)*

H is for HURTS and how to deal with them. It is best to share your feelings instead of assuming that your spouse should know why you are upset. Holding onto hurts clouds the present by nursing unhealed wounds from the past, and blights future communications, causing further pain. Discuss your problems!

'This went on year after year. Whenever Hannah went up to the house of the LORD, her rival provoked her till she wept and would not eat. Elkanah her husband would say to her, "Hannah, why are you weeping? Why don't you eat? Why are you so downhearted . . .?" ' *(1 Samuel 1:7, 8, NIV)*

I is for INTEGRITY.

The deception of lust for power, money and sex can sometimes draw couples apart. Sometimes a sense of dissatisfaction (often irrational) with what one has leads to cravings for something else. This dissatisfaction can compromise the integrity of marriage. Good advice is given in 1 Timothy 6:6: 'But godliness with contentment is great gain.' (NIV)

'Has not the LORD made them one? In flesh and spirit they are his. And why one? Because he was seeking godly offspring. So guard yourself in your spirit, and do not break faith with the wife of your youth.'
(Malachi 2:15, NIV)

I is also for INTEREST.
Keep your interest in each other alive
with the element of surprise. Being
spontaneous brings adventure and
excitement to the marriage. Think of
innovative ways to show interest in your
spouse; it may be something simple like
wearing something new, or a new outfit in
which your spouse desires to see you!

'Your cheeks are beautiful with earrings,
your neck with strings of jewels.'
(Song of Solomon 1:10, NIV)

I

J is for JUGGLING.
Our lives place many
demands on our time. Learning
how to make time for your spouse
among the various competing priorities
is a task in itself. Make sure that neither of
you feels left out or unimportant.

'But Martha was distracted by all the
preparations that had to be made. She
came to him and asked, "Lord, don't you
care that my sister has left me to do the
work by myself? Tell her to help me!"
"Martha, Martha," the Lord answered, "you
are worried and upset about many things,
but only one thing is needed. Mary has
chosen what is better, and it will not be
taken away from her." ' *(Luke 10:40-42, NIV)*

J

K is for KISSES. Kissing increases your levels of oxytocin, a hormone that reduces anxiety and has a significantly calming effect, giving a feeling of peace. Kissing also enhances longevity, as couples who kiss when leaving home in the morning tend to live (on average) five years longer than those who don't.

Kissing is good for the health of your heart as well: adrenaline is released, causing the heart to increase its output of blood around the body.

'Let him kiss me with the kisses of his mouth: for thy love is better than wine'
(Song of Solomon 1:2)

L is for LISTENING. Active listening shows that you are interested in the feelings of your marriage partner as well as the events of your partner's life.

Think of a time when you did this. Can you recall how it made your spouse feel? How would it make you feel? We all like those we love to listen to us, as it affirms us.

'This went on year after year. Whenever Hannah went up to the house of the LORD, her rival provoked her till she wept and would not eat. Elkanah her husband would say to her, "Hannah, why are you weeping? . . ." ' *(1 Samuel 1:7, 8, NIV)*

L is for LOVE. Love is expressed in behaviours, words and decisive actions. Perhaps the best description of love is found in 1 Corinthians 13:4-8:

'Love is patient, love is kind. It does not envy, it does not boast, it is not proud. It is not rude, it is not self-seeking, it is not easily angered, it keeps no record of wrongs. Love does not delight in evil but rejoices with the truth. It always protects, always trusts, always hopes, always perseveres. Love never fails. . . .' *(NIV)*

M is for MONEY MANAGEMENT.
Marriage experts say that differing
attitudes to what one values most come
to the fore when discussing family
finances, causing arguments.

Identify issues like 'income and
expenditure', 'what is affordable and what
isn't', and 'who is the spender and who is
the saver': this will help you work together
towards managing your finances.

'Wisdom is a shelter as money is a shelter,
but the advantage of knowledge is this: that
wisdom preserves the life of its possessor.'
(Ecclesiastes 7:12, NIV)

N is for NURTURE. Holding your spouse close to your heart entails thinking of ways to nurture and build up your spouse. When you invest in each other's well-being, the relationship bond is strengthened. Endearing words and actions, listening attentively, and supporting your spouse in times of challenge can make your spouse feel nurtured.

'His left arm is under my head and his right arm embraces me.'
(Song of Solomon 8:3, NIV)

O is for OBSTACLES.

Sometimes in life, we face obstacles that obscure the beauty of our journey. Identify the stumbling blocks to your relationship: this will help you address issues before they become unmanageable. It also helps you to identify the potential stagnant areas that require work.

'When Rachel saw that she was not bearing Jacob any children, she became jealous of her sister. So she said to Jacob, "Give me children, or I'll die!" '
(Genesis 30:1, NIV)

O is also for OPPORTUNITIES.
Look for opportunities to please your spouse and do something spontaneous as a surprise! Identify what you both want in your marriage; this will give you something to work towards. Many couples now set goals for their marriage, stating the things they want to achieve, both as a couple and as individuals.

'As we have therefore opportunity, let us do good unto all men, especially unto them who are of the household of faith.'
(Galatians 6:10)

O

P is for PATIENCE. No one is perfect – not even you. So be patient towards your spouse, and make allowances. You can both learn from mistakes. Take courage, and move forward together, wiser for the experience.

'Now the God of patience and consolation grant you to be likeminded one toward another according to Christ Jesus'
(Romans 15:5)

P

P is also for PRAYER. Family prayer is by far the most reliable indicator of a long-term satisfying marriage. Couples who pray together have a divorce rate of just 1%, regardless of any other compounding issues.

'Therefore confess your sins to each other and pray for each other so that you may be healed. The prayer of a righteous man is powerful and effective.' *(James 5:16, NIV)*

Q is for QUALITY TIME.
Attentiveness to each other's
needs is enhanced the more time is spent
together. Make time for intimacy; it will pay
dividends now and in the future.

R is for RESPECT. Although this verse refers
to the wife showing respect for her
husband, both the man and the woman
should show respect to each other if the
relationship is to be successful. Never take
each other for granted.

'Nevertheless let each one of you in
particular so love his own wife as himself,
and let the wife see that she respects her
husband.' *(Ephesians 5:33, NKJV)*

R is also for ROMANCE.
Romantic love combines
the elements of care and desire.

'. . . There I will give you my love.'
(Song of Solomon 7:12, NKJV)

S is for SPIRITUALITY. Making God the
Priority in life is life-enhancing. Share
morning and evening worship, prayer and
personal devotion. Growing in Christ
together strengthens the marriage as you
learn to depend on God's guidance.

'But seek first the kingdom of God and His
righteousness, and all these things shall be
added to you.' *(Matthew 6:33, NKJV)*

RS

S is for SEX.

'The husband should fulfill his marital duty to his wife, and likewise the wife to her husband. The wife's body does not belong to her alone but also to her husband. In the same way, the husband's body does not belong to him alone but also to his wife.'
(1 Corinthians 7:3, 4, NIV)

T is for TRUST. This enriches and strengthens marriages. It takes a long time to build, but a short time to destroy. Respect, listen to, and be honest with your spouse; be reliable, articulate your needs, and don't pass on secrets.

U is for UNDERSTANDING.
Alice J. Taylor, when she wrote
that a woman does not ask for her
imperfections to be excused, only that she
be understood, agrees with the psalmist
and King Solomon that understanding is
important: 'Your hands have made me and
fashioned me; Give me understanding, that
I may learn Your commandments.'
(Psalm 119:73, NKJV)

U is for UNITY. You may not always
agree on everything, but being
agreeable is important!

V is for VULNERABILITY.
You must expose your areas
of weakness to your spouse, if
you want your spouse to understand
and support you. This may mean making
yourself vulnerable. It's part of the price we
pay for honest, free, open love.

W is for WELLBEING. Take good care of
yourself – it will pay dividends for both
you and your spouse. Enjoy good
health, good hygiene, stress-relieving
activities and high self-esteem!

'Because of the fragrance of your good
ointments, Your name is ointment poured
forth; Therefore the virgins love you.'
(Song of Solomon 1:3, NKJV)

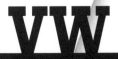

X is for EXTRA SPECIAL.
What is that extra special
'something' that makes your marriage
unique? The special something in Jacob's
marriage to Rachel seems to have been
her beauty: '. . . Rachel was beautiful and
well favoured' *(Genesis 29:17)*

Y is for YOU. As an individual, you are
unique and bring something
special to the relationship.

Z is for ZEST. Ask God to put the zeal
and zest and buzz back into your
relationship so that it becomes exciting
to wake up every day with your
beloved by your side!

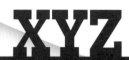

XYZ

AND FINALLY!

The best advice I heard to date
was given on the day Denzle
and I got married.

Unable to attend our wedding, one of my
uncles decided to send a recorded
message for us that could be played at the
reception. Using a baking analogy, my
uncle listed all the ingredients necessary to
bake a good cake, equating them with
various aspects of marriage. He was
careful to point out that the size of the cake
depended on how much of each type of
ingredient was put in. Likewise, in the case
of marriage, the time and effort you
put into it are proportional to the
benefits you may derive from it.

Additionally, when baking,
if one of the ingredients is missing then
the cake will not turn out right: and neither
would a marriage be right if we were to
leave out any of the essential ingredients.

In his conclusion, my uncle said: 'Today,
you have all the necessary ingredients at
your disposal to make the cake you want.'
He advised that we would need to put it
together – it was up to us to do the mixing!
He ended with words with which I
now end and leave you with:
'Go and bake your cake!'